How to Grow Taller

The Ultimate Ways to Increase Your Height Naturally

Allison Lewis

Table of Contents

Introduction

I want to thank you and congratulate you for purchasing the book, *"How to Grow Taller: The Ultimate Ways to Increase Your Height Naturally"*.

Afraid that you will not be employed because of your short height? Done with taller people bullying you at school? Do not worry. This book contains proven steps and strategies on how to increase one's height through natural methods.

This book tells you what to do (and what not to do) in order for you to add inches to your height. Actually, it does not only contain information related to height increase. It enumerates different ideas about height such as superstitious beliefs or myths that people practice until now, bogus ideas about improving your development or growth, and things you might have been doing wrong just to be taller. You may also encounter keywords and learn how are they are related to growth, such a genes, heredity, growth hormone, human ethnic groups (race), and other terminologies.

Do what the book suggests properly and

diligently to notice its full effect. You never know, this book might help you pass height limits and stop bullies from towering against you. It could even help you look at yourself at a completely different (and more positive) way.

Thanks again for purchasing this book, I hope you enjoy it!

Chapter 1 – Uncovering Height

Need extra inches for your height? Are you too short for your job or for your class? Have you tried different things just to get taller but you are still too short?

It is understandable that you might have been doing desperate measures such as believing in superstitious beliefs, praying to deities constantly for your height to grow, and other ways that aren't proven scientifically to height – all because you really want to get taller. Do not worry; this book will help you find answers. After reading this, you'll know a lot more about height. You will discover how to get taller through natural methods that are proven to be effective and beneficial.

Primarily, there are many misconceptions about enhancing height that we still need to clear; fortunately, we will be able to provide you facts concerning your height and how to enhance it. The sheer intention to gain height sometimes waste people's time, as they follow certain beliefs on how to become taller. Other than that, the eagerness also gives shady businesses the opportunity to earn by selling fake, ineffective supplements. This book will show you comparisons between superstition and fact, and pseudoscientific (concepts that may seem to be scientific but turns out otherwise) and scientific concepts.

Fighting Frauds

With matters like this at hand, frauds will be more likely to allure you to buy their products that "guarantee" height growth in no time but do not be a fool to waste your money in such bogus products. Circumstances like these can be considered as very dangerous since there is a low assurance that all of the said ingredients are thoroughly checked and guaranteed to be safe. Some of the used ingredients could lead to an illness or might damage your body internally. Not to mention that, those products are practically unregulated by the FDA.

Studies show that females have already developed their bones once they are at the ages of 16-18, while males fully develop their bones between the ages of 20-21. Therefore, foods and drugs that claim to be able to increase your height will not be able to make you grow once you are in that age because, your height has already reached its limit when your bones are fully developed.

In relation to scammers, take note of the people who claim to be professional and trick you into believing in pseudoscientific claims like, injecting chemicals through your veins to help you boost your height. Simply put, those will not work because the only chemical that involves height is your growth hormone secreted by the pituitary gland, which concerns the bone and not the blood. These kind of bogus people trick their clients with make-believes and gimmicks.

After all procedures have been done and the clients have settled their accounts, these fake professionals run away before the said clients complain about the tremendous side effects and devastating results. Those pseudoscientific methods that have been done may lead to damage towards the blood, heart, brain or it may possibly lead to death.

Understanding Myths

Myths, on the other hand, point out that man cannot acquire Osteoporosis but in fact, men who are aged 50 and above are at risk and can acquire this bone disease. It is just that Osteoporosis among men is overlooked and unrecorded. There are many myths about height growth in different cultures.

Some even believe that jumping during New Year's Eve at exactly twelve o'clock will make you grow taller the coming year. During New year this is still practiced by believers who want to be taller but we all know that there are no proven explanation that this is effective enough to make you grow taller.

Looking Into Science

Research has revealed that height depends on genetics, diet, activities and environment. Other than that, people of science have already given us facts like how our height differs during sleep because the backbone's size slightly increases. Auxology, the study of human growth, states that stature or height is sexually dimorphic, which means that certain traits are different from each gender. In other words, the typical male height differs from the average female height, mainly due to differences in leg length and proportion.

Also, from the previous statement, the years where the bones of males develop are much longer than those of females. This translates to a higher possibility for men to be taller than women do. Auxology also shows that certain defects that are correlated to height (such as Gigantism) are only acquired by those individuals who have hyperpituitarism, wherein the pituitary gland secretes too much growth hormone. There are some cases also wherein the pituitary gland secretes growth hormones slower than normal. This may result to Dwarfism or Idiopathic Short Stature.

Chapter 2 – Genes and You

Before we discuss further about naturally increasing our height, we must first explore the world of human genes, gene recombination, and how those things affect height.

The word "Genes" came from the ancient Greek word" *genos*" meaning "race or offspring". Genes are special units of DNA which also manipulate traits that may be inherited from generation to generation. The discovery of Genes was due to a Gregorian monk's simple experiment of inheritance. This discovery resulted to the conclusion of the possibility of parents' traits being passed down to their offspring.

Height traits, however, unlike other common traits, is considered to be very complicated to understand or to predict especially when genetic recombination is present. Genetic recombination refers to product genes having neither trait from the parents, meaning the genes have completely combined the parents' traits that none of the distinctive quality of the parents is seen in the offspring. For example, having a short parent and tall parent may result to an average-height child.

An ethnic group, as defined in sociology, is determined by both cultural similarities and cultural differences. An ethnic group may consist of blood-related human beings or people who follow the same norm. Some researchers predict that within cultural groups, the possibility of an individual mating with another individual within his or her ethnic group is very high. Due to that repetitive event, researchers speculate that, no matter how big a cultural group may be, members have the possibility of being blood related. This created patterns on the different features a certain group has.

It was believed that the patterns of growth vary within different ethnic groups. It is believed that the succeeding generations in different cultural groups are not only affected by the blood composition of the ancestral generation, but also by the practices done by one's ancestors.

As proof of the previous statements, according to research, people coming from the African-Caribbean regions are much taller and heavier, while Asian and Chinese groups are shorter and lighter unlike Caucasians (white people with European origin). More recently, a study group disproved this belief, implying that being born within the population can promise a high possibility of being taller than living in a different place with different norms. It is just that African-Caribbean groups are known for ship work and manpower. They are known to do things manually, like, carrying things by group, or simply finishing tasks by the use of their bare hands. Since these actions are done repetitively, children within this group has a high chance of maximizing the genes of their parents.

A Direct Connection

Height itself involves our genes. Other studies mention that approximately 75% of our height came from the blueprint of life (DNA) while the other 25% can be affected by environmental factors, which includes habitual actions, and favorable surroundings. Studies show that 80% of people in a certain population have gene-determined height, while the remaining 20% of people obtained their height due to their environment. Therefore, we can say that your height does not rely on genetics alone. Another fanciful point about genes is that, today's biologists are working on accurate prediction of one's offspring's height.

Increasing height naturally may be hard for some people. Genetic composition may be difficult to change but, if we just work hard and smart, we will surely achieve our desired height. In the next chapters, factors that affect the height of individuals living in different societies, having different beliefs, and exercising different practices, will be discussed. Along with the affecting factors are the natural methods that we suggest, which are flexible enough to be applicable to any person that aspires to become taller without spending too much time.

Chapter 3 – Diet and Its Impact

A factor that might increase your height naturally is diet, since getting more nutrients involved in digestion and bone development can definitely help. China constantly advised individuals to eat food that is more nutritious. As a result, the common height in China increased by roughly six inches. Meanwhile, other countries that lack good nourishing food or are being plagued by malnutrition, have shorter individuals.

A meal or diet plan is defined as the organization of the amount of food intake, types of food that shall be ingested, and the time in which the food prepared will be eaten. A diet plan may be made daily, weekly, monthly, or even annually. Most people do meal planning in order to maintain a healthy diet or to achieve certain goals or objectives. In order for a diet plan/meal plan to be effective, one must first analyze his or her body. You must first understand how your system works, so that you could follow a diet plan that is suitable for your needs. It would be better if you analyze this with a dietician (an expert in human nutrition).

Many people nowadays prefer searching through the World Wide Web for meal plans rather than walking to a clinic to consult a specialist personally. Commonly, the meal plans found on the web are based on the different food groups. Food groups refer to classified food having biological similarities. There are five common food groups, namely the dairy group, the fruit group, the grain foods, the lean meats and poultry, fish, eggs, tofu, nuts and seeds group, and the vegetables, legumes, and beans group.

Focusing on what's Important

In the dairy group, we would find the foods rich in calcium. Calcium is important for a person to have strong and healthy bones. Most foods that belong to other groups do not contain as much calcium compared those in the dairy group. The fruit group is where we find foods that are rich in vitamins, minerals, and other nutrients that could help in the growth and development of the body.

The grain foods, also known as the "cereal group" or "carbohydrates group", are where we find foods that are rich in carbohydrates. Some foods that belong in this group may be high in sugar, fat, and sodium.

The fourth group, also known as the "lean meats and poultry, fish, eggs, tofu, nuts, and seeds group" is where we find foods that are rich in protein, which is essential for height increase. The vegetables, legumes, and beans group is the group where we also find foods rich in vitamins, minerals, and other nutrients crucial to the development of the body.

There are a lot of food containing the vitamins and minerals needed for growth such as milk and fish (both milk and fish belong to the "grow foods", which is a food group known for their protein content) which both contain calcium – the building blocks of bones. Insufficient calcium intake could result to Osteoporosis and Calcium Deficiency (hypocalcaemia). Milk and Fish are also rich in Vitamin D, which improves Calcium absorption in the bones. Vitamin D plays a role in balancing hormones as well. Lack of this Vitamin can lead to *rickets* (disease of having soft or weak bones) and bone deformity. Foods like fish and milk are also rich in Vitamin B12 or the so-called *riboflavin,* which helps stimulate bone development.

Spinach is a food rich in vitamins and minerals, particularly those that could affect height. Magnesium, for one, helps maintain bone density (the strength of bones) by concentrating calcium towards the bones. Lack of Magnesium causes Hypocalcaemia. Spinach also has Potassium, which makes the body more alkaline. The body needs to avoid being acidic and if it is, your body will signal your bones to breakdown parts of it to balance out the acid-base levels.

Phosphorus is also present in Spinach, and it's known to help maintain bone health. In addition to that, Spinach contains many proteins, which help in keeping the bone structure whole. This special kind of food also has Vitamin A, needed to synthesize protein.

Foods such as chocolate, oyster, and peas are rich in Zinc, which plays a role in maintaining bone health. A child who does not have enough Zinc tends to have abnormal or below-average height.

Rice and Pork are important sources of Vitamin B1, which is needed for growth and proper digestion. As you might notice, most of the said vitamins and minerals are for bone health. It is because bone growth is intimately related to height. Remember that maintaining healthy bones means increasing your height.

Not only should we keep track of our food intake, but also of the amount of water that we drink throughout the day. Research suggests that on average, humans must be able to drink six to eight glasses of water. Water intake does not only replenish our body, but it also boosts the effects of the vitamins, minerals, and other nutrients that we take in order to have an increase in height.

A Vital Reminder

At this point, you are probably thinking of filling your fridge with the food mentioned in this chapter. You might be planning to solely rely on them for nourishment. Well, that's not wise thing to do. Always check whether your dietary plans match what health experts recommend. This may help you decide on what meal you can have next, and it can help you become conscious of the amount you eat. Try to integrate the foods listed here into properly portioned dishes and nutritionally balanced meal plans.

Chapter 4 – Advantageous Activities

Activities could also naturally improve your height without the use of anything fancy. Activities that involve increasing your height relates to stretching your bones most, especially your vertebra, when they have fully developed. Methods that involve correcting your posture and stretching your muscles vertically can greatly contribute to increasing your height.

The most common exercise known to gradually increase height is stretching, which involves flexing your muscle's growing points to enable growth. Stretching can be subdivided into seven types namely:

- Ballistic

- Isometric

- PNF (Proprioceptive Neuromuscular Facilitation)

- Dynamic

- Active

- Passive

- Static

Take note that Ballistic, Isometric, and PNF stretching involves your body's momentum, forcing you to reach your limit in speed and endurance. The three stated stretches are stretches that are not recommended; therefore, they should be avoided by anyone who wishes to gain height. They are also too extensive for people who are still developing their bones, such as kids and adolescents. Why? It is mainly due to their greater-than-usual flexibility in the joints and bones, meaning extensive stretches could lead to connective-tissue damage.

On the other hand, Dynamic stretches are exercises that include controlled arm and leg swing motions, which are performed more gently compared to Ballistic stretches. Active stretching is about holding a stretched position for the longest time you can do, for example, holding your leg up for 30 seconds or more. Active stretches are done without any help while passive stretching requires an apparatus or assistance from an object or partner. For instance, doing the splits on the floor helps you sustain your extended form. The floor played as an apparatus in this instant. When holding your knee up with the help of your hand, the hand plays the role of the apparatus.

Static and Passive stretches are closely similar. The only difference is that, Static stretching is stretching to the farthest but it does not necessarily require an apparatus and does not involve any movement.

Doing basic stretches, such as sit and reach or bridge stretch, can also do the trick. Still, to gain the full benefit of stretching, you must execute stretches at least 15 minutes a day. Another way to stretch your spines and joints is by staying upside down. Here, you will defy gravity (which actually hinders us to grow taller and compresses our body downwards). You can easily do this on a monkey bar or anything that can lift your weight above the ground, do this constantly to have a difference with regards to your height.

There are simpler ways to increase your height, such as skipping rope. It does not just help you become slimmer, as it also helps your calf muscle extend vertically. Furthermore, skipping forces your muscles to stretch and contract (especially the tendons and ligaments), making them more flexible. Skipping rope also helps in elongating your bones. In addition to that, when you skip rope, you stand taller, decompressing your spine and correcting your posture.

Power of Slumber

Usually, doctors and other health professionals would recommend a good night's sleep for a healthier body, which is taken as fact because adequate sleep also contributes in human growth. Specialists have proven that during sleep, your height is altered because your backbone relaxes and slightly extends. Other than that, having eight hours of sleep is enough time for your body to regenerate and to enable your brain to relax and slow down. As a result, the pituitary gland efficiently works on the secretion of growth hormone. Therefore, the longer you sleep, the higher the chance that growth hormones are released in your body.

As to be expected, sleep deprivation may cause stunted growth, due to the lack of growth hormone.

Swimming Solution

Health analysts have also found out that swimming is one of the best activities for enhancing your height because it involves your hands and feet doing things simultaneously. The best style for improving your height is said to be the breaststroke, which requires your hands to strike from the breast to the sides in full lengths at both directions and your feet to paddle in one direction. This results to stretching your spine and muscles. In addition, it helps in stimulating the production of growth hormone, as swimming boosts the production of two important components needed for growth hormone secretion, namely lactate and nitric oxide. Research also shows that kids who habitually swim are more likely to grow taller than those who are non-swimmers.

Consider Doing Yoga

Another healthy activity for height improvement is Yoga. Although it does not help in bone growth, it helps in stretching your spine by correcting your posture and spine endurance. Some of the methods used in Yoga that will help you grow taller are the *Ardha Kurmasana* and *Bhujangasana*.

Ardha Kurmasana is also known as the "half tortoise pose". It is done by bending your knees on the floor and arching your back towards your knees, so that your chest and knees are kept close to each other while you extend your arms in front, with both palms closed, facing each other. This posture should look like a tortoise when performed. This posture helps you avoid back pain and spinal problems. Furthermore, it also elongates your spine.

Bhujangasana which is known as the "snake pose" is executed by laying both feet on the floor and raising your head and torso upwards, then slightly bending backwards leaving both feet to lay on the floor. *Bhujangasana* increases spine flexibility, strength, and length.

Ponder on Pilates

Pilates is one of the most known extensive power core exercises, which also help in boosting growth, just like Yoga. It does not help in increasing the size of bones but it extends the backbone. Pilate is a group of exercises mainly for core (referring to the muscles located from your back to the abdomen) strength. One routine in Pilates is the *Pilates Hundreds*. This is done by bending your knees, keeping your feet on the floor while you curl your head and shoulders; you are your lower back still pressed to the floor. Then, you will have to put your arms at the side of your hip and slightly pump them up and down. This helps you in strengthening your spine, as well as in enhancing its endurance.

On Things to Avoid

In order to gain positive results, you should avoid doing certain things. Activities such as smoking, which deteriorates the cells needed for growth hormones to be secreted. It is also recommended to avoid drinking alcohol in excessive amounts. Too much alcohol greatly damages the liver. By the way, smoking damages the liver as well. The liver plays an important role in the production of protein, which is needed by the bones. Without it, sustaining the bone structure can be difficult.

One of the things to avoid while you are trying to add inches to your height is having extensive workouts and weight lifting, because doing these might confuse your body and force it to concentrate on muscle development. Nevertheless, increasing your height requires light exercises to fully relax, stretch your backbone, and to keep a good posture. When an individual is stressed, he/she is capable of producing bad hormones, which may negatively affect the body's different cycles. That is why reducing stress is highly advised because it not only helps with regards to your vertebra, but, it also helps in ensuring efficient Human Growth Hormone production.

Chapter 5 – Environment's Role

The type of environment a person lives in can affect height. If we observe closely, people who live in urbanized areas tend to be taller compared to the people who live in the rural areas.

In addition, some researchers say that the socio-economic status of an individual greatly affects the probability of increasing height through natural ways, but some say otherwise. People just have to be creative enough to look for an alternative when the resources are not available.

Humans have established communities and flourished around sources of clean, potable water and fresh air since the beginning of time. It is vital to our survival and growth. Air pollution can gravely affect our health and disrupt our body systems, which may hinder growth. Almost everything that is a byproduct of our civilization is polluting our drinking water and surrounding air. Drinking polluted and unclean water can greatly damage your digestive tract. Infectious diseases can be spread through contaminated water or even from the dirty atmosphere. Airborne and waterborne diseases have a big impact on height.

Now, the question is, how can we increase our height despite living in polluted environments? We just need to be cautious.

Drinking clean water could help vitamins and minerals, have a greater effect on our body. We must practice good sanitation when we are preparing food to protect our immune system, and prevent diseases that may affect our stature. It is because diseases reduce the body's capacity for growth. Remember that, a safe and natural environment, and a healthy lifestyle, increases our chances of increasing our height.

Living in a wholesome environment can greatly affect your height because, partly, your height depends on the environment you are living in. The environment enables factors that greatly influence your height. An environment that enables you to do activities for your height without any disturbance, a place where you can practice yoga peacefully, can increase the probability of you becoming taller.

Likewise, a pollution-free environment may help your brain be at ease so that your pituitary gland may work better. A smoke- and alcohol-free environment is also of great help, especially when it comes to avoiding growth deficiency. Other than that, having the right environment for sleep is necessary for a person to increase their height, due to the importance of undisturbed sleep during growth. Lastly, an environment wherein you have access to foods rich in vitamins and minerals needed for growth will allow you to nourish your bones and muscles.

Learning from History

The Nilotic people (Indigenous people who majorly inhabit Southern Sudan) are described to have long legs and narrow bodies, which create the image of being tall. The said distinct features were further explained by researchers as something these individuals possess due to the need to adapt to hot weather.

Nilotic people can be further divided into several groups. Two of those groups are the *Shilluk and Dinka,* wherein the average height of the people of *Shilluk* that were recorded was 5 feet and 11 inches. Meanwhile, the average height of the people of *Dinka* that was recorded was approximately 6 feet. This was before wars began to break out. However, after the wars, the remaining refugees were again measured, and resulted to a change of their average height, which is now 5 feet and 6-7 inches. A probable explanation for this was that the war hindered them from getting enough nourishment and rest.

Aside from the Nilotic people the children in Guatemala have also manifested this sudden change. This was noticed by Barry Bogin who conducted his studies in the early 1970s. He took note their average height. During the Guatemalan Civil war, the Guatemala Maya children fled to the United States of America. Soon, after the war, he again measured the height of average children aged 6-12 and noticed that the results were higher than those gathered before the war began. This is because these refugees were able to get proper nourishment, in an environment that enabled their growth.

These two mentioned studies are concrete proof that the environment is able to manipulate height and can either sustain it or change it. This was obviously manifested in both cases. Therefore, the environment and individual growth are distinctly correlated. As for their relevance to you, aside from highlighting the need to stay in an environment that supports growth, you need to stay away from those that could essentially hamper your body's development – you need to move away from places stress you out continuously and considerably.

Chapter 6 – A Quick Summary

As implied throughout the previous chapters, height is a distinct feature that humans possess but, in a typical person's point of view, it is either being short or being tall. Height itself is a classic feature yet it is a very complicated concept. People who find their height to be far from beneficial tend to find ways to change their stature. Some believe in myths and other traditions concerning height growth, and practice them. For some, they search for proven methods in order to have their desired height. Giving time and effort to grow taller is worth it. You just need to understand the variables that affect your growth and focus on them.

Having tall parents may give you bigger chances of being tall, but if you're short even at this situation, then you can enhance your height by eating the said foods such milk, fish, egg, spinach, meat, chocolates, and rice – these boost bone development due to the great amounts of vitamins and minerals they contain, like Protein, Calcium, Vitamin D, Magnesium, Zinc, Vitamin B1, Vitamin B6, Vitamin C, and Phosphorus. Any food containing these vitamins and minerals is good for an individual's body as long as it is eaten in appropriate amounts. Having too much might not be helpful.

If you want to be tall and active, try stretching at least 15 minutes a day, hanging on a bar for like 2-3 minutes a day, or skipping rope which may be helpful because it elongates your legs and corrects your posture. Correcting your posture helps you in decompressing your spine which can make you taller. This can be done through yoga, Pilates, swimming, and other outdoor activities that can bend, stretch, and relax your backbone, but remember not to overdo it nor execute extensive activities because it might lead to injury.

Pushing yourself too hard can stress you, increasing the production of bad hormones that disrupt your body's cycle. Lastly, the most important method to be done to increase your height is sleeping. It does not only relax your vertebra but it also helps in the secretion of growth hormones.

You must also take note that to become taller, you need to live in a favorable environment where growth can be supported. This environment must be able to let you sleep and do activities you'd like in peace, able to provide what you need for nourishment. And of course, a pollution-free environment helps a lot in your growth process.

Height is a distinctive feature depend on genetics, diet, activity, and environment.

Doing what has been said in this book might earn you a credit for giving your time and effort for a healthier body. Remember that your height is not the sole factor in determining how desirable you are because at the end of the day, the things you do will define you.

Conclusion

Thank you again for purchasing this book!

I hope this book was able to help you acquire the necessary information on how to increase your height through natural methods.

The next step is to try the different things that may help you create a difference in your height. Always remember that you are the master of your own body.

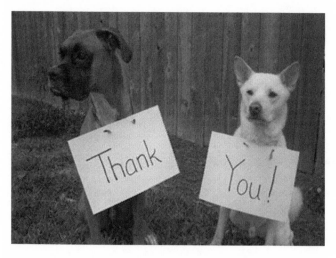

Finally, if you enjoyed this book, then I would like to ask you for a favor, would you be kind enough to leave a review for this book on Amazon? It'd be greatly appreciated!

Thank you and good luck!

Made in the USA
Las Vegas, NV
04 March 2024

86693183R00021